Functional Fitness

Building a Strong Foundation for Everyday Life

(The Essential Guide to Optimal Firefighter Performance and Longevity)

Joshua Foster

Published By **Kate Sanders**

Joshua Foster

All Rights Reserved

Functional Fitness: Building a Strong Foundation for Everyday Life (The Essential Guide to Optimal Firefighter Performance and Longevity)

ISBN 978-1-7777621-2-4

No part of this guidebook shall be reproduced in any form without permission in writing from the publisher except in the case of brief quotations embodied in critical articles or reviews.

Legal & Disclaimer

The information contained in this book is not designed to replace or take the place of any form of medicine or professional medical advice. The information in this book has been provided for educational & entertainment purposes only.

The information contained in this book has been compiled from sources deemed reliable, and it is accurate to the best of the Author's knowledge; however, the Author cannot guarantee its accuracy and validity and cannot be held liable for any errors or omissions. Changes are periodically made to this book. You must consult your doctor or get professional medical advice before using any of the suggested remedies, techniques, or information in this book.

Table Of Contents

Chapter 1: The Foundation of Functional Longevity

In the pursuit of placing up with properly-being and a life filled with energy, this chapter unfurls the profound interconnection between sensible education and longevity. Positioned as a foundational cornerstone, it lays the premise for next discussions, emphasizing the imperative function that beneficial schooling performs in retaining physical independence, promoting holistic properly being, and fostering highbrow acuity throughout the spectrum of lifestyles.

1.1 Exploring the Interplay amongst Functional Training and Longevity:

Beyond the mere extension of chronological existence, functional sturdiness emerges as a qualitative organization that seeks to optimize each factor of our life. This segment delves into the symbiosis among realistic schooling and durability, casting slight on its transformative potential for people of each age.

1. Holistic Wellness: Beyond the confines of conventional health metrics, sensible longevity embraces a holistic ethos. It aspires now not simply to increase existence but to supplement it, safeguarding important factors which include mobility, flexibility, and intellectual well-being. The narrative unfolds a imaginative and prescient wherein well-being isn't always compartmentalized however

as a substitute, an interconnected tapestry of physical and intellectual energy.

2. Adaptable Fitness across Age Groups: The adaptability of practical education emerges as a unifying situation count, making it an inclusive platform resonating with people at some point of severa age companies. From seniors seeking out to make stronger balance and mobility to more youthful fans laying the inspiration for future properly-being, functional training will become a flexible and to be had health philosophy.

1.2 Benefits of Prioritizing Functional Movements for Long-Term Health:

Within this subsection, we embark on a nuanced exploration of the precise blessings that prioritizing functional movements bestows upon prolonged-time period health and electricity.

1. Joint Health: The tough relationship amongst realistic moves and joint fitness is unveiled. By aligning with herbal movement patterns, beneficial wearing activities become an instrumental tool in promoting joint flexibility, mitigating the effect of developing vintage, and fostering popular musculoskeletal resilience.

2. Cognitive Well-Being: The financial disaster delves deep into the cognitive blessings inherent in practical education. Beyond physical prowess, useful moves have interaction the mind, imparting a holistic approach to maintaining intellectual sharpness and agility. The interconnectedness of

bodily and cognitive properly-being emerges as a cornerstone for a satisfying and enduring existence.

3. Independence in Daily Living: As life progresses through its diverse ranges, the importance of maintaining independence in every day sports will become paramount. This phase underscores how realistic training cultivates the vital abilties required for navigating each day responsibilities with autonomy and self-reliance.

4. Long-Term Sustainability: The narrative on the enduring nature of purposeful training is stepped forward further, positioning it now not clearly as a temporary fashion however as a lifelong accomplice in the pursuit of sensible longevity. The sustainability of practical carrying sports over the

long term turns into a defining element in their effectiveness, underscoring the significance of a health philosophy that withstands the take a look at of time.

As we draw the curtain in this foundational financial disaster, the complicated dance between beneficial schooling and sturdiness comes into sharper popularity. The standards laid out right right here cross past traditional fitness paradigms, championing a holistic technique that resonates with people at each degree of lifestyles. This chapter sets the volume for a whole exploration of strategies beneficial education intertwines with the vital additives of durability. By delving into the holistic advantages, adaptability, and enduring nature of beneficial actions, it propels us right into a multifaceted adventure closer to sustained properly-being across the complete spectrum of existence.

Chapter 2: Functional Training

Ever perplexed about the ones fitness guides you have got stumble upon? Let's damage down practical education. Imagine it as the call of the game sauce for your normal movements, like sitting, reputation, carrying out for stuff, or perhaps pulling a automobile – all inspired by means of way of the usage of sporting activities like squats, presses, and pulls.

Functional health is shape of a chameleon, becoming into your day anytime, anywhere, and in any outfit. Whether you are into easy frame weight sports activities or spicing matters up with cool adjustable dumbbells and stretchy bands, getting equipped for practical power education is your fee price ticket to building muscles and boosting your coronary heart health.

"Functional training is not quite tons the gym," says the professional. "Nowadays, it is all about the use of bands, balls, ropes, kettlebells, sandbags, or maybe tires to get your frame transferring specially methods."

Picture beneficial education as a teamwork of muscle mass and joints — like a squat, in which your hips, knees, and ankles gracefully bend and straighten. Your essential muscle game enthusiasts, the glutes and quads, lead the display, with supporting roles from the hamstrings, calves, and erector spinae (they've got your once more — truely). And we've no longer even referred to your middle muscular tissues stepping up to the plate!

Functional education is like an art work shape outside the gymnasium, inviting you to create a balanced dance of electricity and versatility to your frame.

2.1. Core Principles of Functional Training

Functional schooling, regularly misconstrued, extends a long way beyond the usage of gymnasium gadget in unconventional ways. It is ready replicating moves inherent for your enterprise or each day lifestyles. This bankruptcy delves into the center requirements that underpin beneficial schooling, providing a foundation for a holistic technique to health.

Defining Functional Training:

At its essence, beneficial training isn't always pretty much physical movements; it is a technique that strengthens and conditions particular mechanical and active characteristics of the human frame, aligning them with a centered outcome. These standards are channeled through 4 pillars: locomotion, degree changes, push and pull, and rotation.

Exploring Locomotion:

Irrespective of your interest, movement from point A to B is essential. Whether it entails skipping, leaping, sidestepping, or sprinting, single-leg moves take priority. This section demanding conditions the conventional use of squats and introduces the single-leg anterior attain as a extra sensible opportunity.

Navigating Level Changes:

From low to immoderate, the dynamics of movement alternate significantly. Staggered deadlifts, differing from the parallel stance of conventional deadlifts, turn out to be a beneficial choice whilst getting up from a fall or lifting an item. Using dumbbells or cables to vary the increase attitude complements the functionality of these exercises.

Engaging in Push and Pull Movements:

In each day life, pushing and pulling movements predominantly get up at the same time as status, necessitating engagement of the middle and precise muscle organizations. The financial disaster advises on sensible alternatives, suggesting repute cable presses over the traditional bench press for pushing strength and highlighting the effectiveness of bent-over rows as a superior practical pulling go with the flow in assessment to pull-ups.

Mastering Rotation:

Rotation needs a twin method—acceleration and deceleration all through sports sports sports activities sports like walking or twisting. Developing rotational strength requires no longer handiest movement however moreover middle stiffness. Traditional center wearing sports can also fall quick, and the financial ruin recommends twisting wearing sports the usage of resistance bands or cables. A favourite, the band or cable rotation, is unique as an awesome approach for developing center energy with a dual-reason consciousness.

2.2: Types of Functional Exercises for Comprehensive Fitness

Building upon the middle ideas mentioned inside the preceding segment, Chapter 2.2 explores various types of useful sports activities activities tailor-made for entire fitness. These wearing activities are designed to decorate no longer handiest particular muscle organizations but also regular capability, selling a properly-rounded technique to physical nicely-being.

Dynamic Movement Patterns:

Functional bodily games are first rate via their capacity to duplicate actual-world moves. This phase delves into dynamic movement styles that interact multiple muscle groups simultaneously. Exercises like medicinal drug ball slams, woodchoppers, and kettlebell swings are explored for their efficacy in fostering coordination, power, and versatility.

Bodyweight Functional Training:

Functional health is not reliant on outside weights. This part highlights the importance of body weight sports activities activities, emphasizing movements that leverage your very very own body for resistance. Squats, lunges, push-ups, and planks are tested as fundamental body weight sporting sports activities that make contributions to commonplace electricity, stability, and staying electricity.

Balance and Stability Exercises:

Balance is a critical aspect of beneficial fitness, especially for seniors or the ones aiming to enhance balance. This section introduces bodily video video games which includes single-leg stands, balance ball sports activities, and balance board sports. These bodily video video games no longer simplest enhance stability but also interact middle muscle groups, contributing to traditional stability.

Functional Training with Resistance Bands:

Resistance bands offer a bendy technique to functional training. They provide adjustable resistance degrees and can be effects included into various physical sports activities. This part explores bodily sports like band pull-aparts, lateral walks, and resisted rotations, showcasing how resistance bands beautify muscle engagement and joint balance.

Agility and Speed Drills:

Functional fitness is going beyond strength; it encompasses agility and speed. Agility ladder drills, cone drills, and dash versions are mentioned to demonstrate how incorporating the ones sporting activities can decorate now not handiest cardiovascular health however moreover beautify agility and quickness in every day sports.

Integrated Functional Workouts:

The financial ruin concludes by illustrating the way to integrate remarkable varieties of practical physical video video games into entire workout workout routines. Sample exercising physical activities are supplied, showcasing the aggregate of dynamic movements, frame weight physical video games, stability drills, resistance band education, and agility drills to create a properly-rounded and powerful functional fitness ordinary.

This phase dreams to equip readers with a severa repertoire of useful sports activities activities, offering a holistic technique to fitness that targets various factors of bodily nicely-being.

Chapter 3: Strength Training Recommendations

In Chapter 3, we delve into the essential realm of electricity training inside the context of useful health. Understanding the importance of energy is paramount for not unusual functionality, and this chapter offers suggestions to tailor strength training to person desires and skills.

Importance of Strength Training:

Strength is the foundation of practical health. This section emphasizes the significance of strength schooling in enhancing muscle mass, bone density, and common physical resilience. From enhancing every day activities to stopping accidents, the blessings of incorporating electricity education into your habitual are explored.

Functional Strength vs. Traditional Approaches:

Differentiating purposeful electricity from traditional strategies is crucial. The bankruptcy compares sensible electricity, emphasizing actual-world programs, with traditional energy education techniques. It highlights the importance of appealing more than one muscle organizations concurrently to imitate the desires of every day lifestyles.

Tailoring Strength Training:

One length does not match all in electricity education. This element gives steerage on tailoring power training physical games to man or woman needs and abilties. Whether you are a amateur or an professional fitness enthusiast, know-how your frame and frequently developing intensity is key to a sustainable and effective energy training application.

Functional Core Strength:

A robust center is important to beneficial health. This segment explores bodily video games especially designed to bolster the middle in strategies that guide traditional capability. Planks, anti-rotation bodily video video games, and dynamic center movements are discussed to offer a nicely-rounded method to constructing practical center energy.

Functional Movements for Everyday Activities:

The financial ruin showcases electricity training sports activities that without delay translate into progressed overall performance in every day sports. From lifting groceries to transferring furnishings, beneficial actions collectively with squats, deadlifts, and farmer's consists of are dissected to awareness on their relevance in enhancing each day capability.

Adapting for Different Fitness Levels:

Fitness is a journey, and it's miles essential to conform power schooling to particular fitness levels. This element gives changes and progressions for severa physical sports, making sure that human beings at awesome stages in their fitness journey can interact in powerful and constant electricity education tailor-made to their capabilities.

Progressive Overload for Functional Strength:

Progressive overload is a critical principle in power education. This section explores how little by little developing resistance, amount, or intensity is vital for chronic development. By regularly tough your muscle groups, you sell ongoing variations, main to sustained profits in practical energy.

Balancing Muscular Imbalances:

Functional power necessitates a balanced development of muscle groups to prevent imbalances that could cause accidents. The economic disaster delves into strategies for addressing and correcting muscular imbalances, emphasizing the importance of concentrated on opposing muscle groups and addressing weaknesses to foster famous purposeful symmetry.

Functional Strength in Aging:

As we age, maintaining useful strength turns into increasingly more vital. This thing discusses how electricity education tailor-made to the wishes of older adults can beautify mobility, bone density, and fashionable power. Exercises that specialize in beneficial moves and joint flexibility are highlighted to aid healthy growing vintage.

Incorporating Functional Strength into Workouts:

The effectiveness of strength training lies in its integration into entire exercise workouts. This phase gives sensible insights into seamlessly incorporating beneficial strength carrying activities into various exercise plans. Whether you select complete-body exercises or specific muscle commercial enterprise agency targeted on, the bankruptcy offers steering on growing a nicely-rounded electricity training ordinary.

Recovery Strategies for Strength Training:

Recovery is a essential detail of any strength education software program. This element explores strategies to optimize restoration, together with proper nutrients, good enough sleep, and targeted stretching. Understanding the significance of recuperation not extremely good enhances the effectiveness of power education but also prevents burnout and decreases the risk of injuries.

Monitoring and Adjusting Strength Training Programs:

No strength education software program is static. Regular evaluation and adjustment are key to long-time period fulfillment. This phase outlines the manner to screen improvement, come to be aware of regions for development, and make critical adjustments to make certain ongoing effectiveness and save you plateaus in useful strength development.

three.1 Importance of Strength Training for Overall Functionality

In this segment, we delve into the cornerstone of useful health—

strength education. Understanding the paramount significance of energy in the realm of general functionality is top to unlocking a resilient, agile, and strong body able to assembly the demands of regular lifestyles.

Foundational Pillar of Functionality:

Strength is the bedrock upon which all sensible motion styles relaxation. Whether lifting, pushing, pulling, or without a doubt navigating the stressful situations of each day sports, a robust basis of power underpins every movement. This detail elucidates how electricity serves due to the fact the critical building block for vast capability.

Enhanced Muscle Mass and Metabolism:

Strength education is going beyond the right away earnings in muscle power; it contributes extensively to advanced muscle mass. More muscle agencies now not fantastic elevates basal metabolic charge however furthermore complements the body's capability to burn power at relaxation. This segment explores how energy schooling, by means of the use of manner of fostering muscle growth, performs a pivotal feature in keeping a healthy frame composition.

Bone Health and Density:

The significance of power schooling extends to the skeletal gadget. Weight-bearing bodily activities stimulate bone formation and decorate bone density. This is particularly important in preventing osteoporosis and promoting wellknown bone fitness. The financial ruin information the characteristic of strength education in fortifying the skeletal form, ensuring sturdiness and resilience.

Joint Stability and Injury Prevention:

Functional movement is based on the steadiness of joints. Strength training goals the muscle tissues surrounding joints, presenting crucial manual and stability. By reinforcing those structures, people are higher organized to prevent accidents and navigate each day sports with decreased danger. This element emphasizes the symbiotic relationship among energy training, joint stability, and harm prevention.

Improving Functional Capacity:

Strength is the linchpin for growing purposeful capability. From the capacity to hold groceries to the ability for unbiased living, power education without delay correlates with advanced functionality. The monetary catastrophe explores how focused power wearing occasions translate into extra appropriate widespread performance in every day sports activities, fostering independence and satisfactory of life.

Mitigating the Impact of Aging:

Aging frequently accompanies a natural decline in muscle groups and power. Strength training emerges as a excellent countermeasure. This section highlights how incorporating electricity bodily games into one's regular can mitigate the effect of developing older, maintaining muscular tissues, bone density, and regular functionality properly into the later degrees of lifestyles.

Holistic Impact on Mental Health:

Beyond the bodily blessings, strength schooling exerts a remarkable have an impact on on intellectual well-being. This element explores the mental elements, discussing how the feel of accomplishment, stepped forward arrogance, and the discharge of endorphins make a contribution to a holistic enhancement of mental health via strength training.

Functional Independence:

Strength training lays the idea for sensible independence. This phase explores how building electricity in severa muscle businesses right now interprets into the functionality to carry out every day obligations without reliance on outside assist. From mountaineering stairs to lifting gadgets, the energy received via targeted sports activities empowers human beings to hold autonomy in their sports sports.

Preventing Chronic Conditions:

The advantages of energy schooling expand to preventing chronic situations. Maintaining muscular energy is related to a discounted threat of chronic ailments collectively with diabetes, cardiovascular troubles, and weight issues. By actively undertaking electricity schooling, human beings contribute to their long-term health and properly-being, stopping the onset of debilitating situations.

Enhanced Posture and Body Mechanics:

A sturdy musculoskeletal device, fostered via strength education, without a doubt influences posture and body mechanics. This element delves into the relationship among muscular electricity and proper alignment, elucidating how electricity education aids in keeping proper posture and gold desired frame mechanics. Improved alignment, in flip, reduces the danger of musculoskeletal problems.

Empowering Functional Longevity:

The segment concludes by way of emphasizing how electricity schooling is a key participant in empowering useful durability. As human beings age, the upkeep of strength becomes a linchpin for maintaining an lively and nice lifestyles. Strength education emerges as a dependable accomplice on the adventure closer to not clearly durability but a lifestyles characterised via power and the capacity to consist of latest disturbing situations.

3.2: Tailoring Strength Training to Individual Needs and Abilities

In this phase, we navigate the nuanced terrain of tailoring energy schooling to individual dreams and skills. Recognizing that a one-length-suits-all method might not be finest, this bankruptcy explores how customization can enhance the effectiveness and sustainability of power education for diverse human beings.

Understanding Individual Goals:

The cornerstone of tailoring electricity schooling lies in know-how man or woman dreams. This element delves into the importance of clarifying personal goals, whether or not or no longer they revolve round muscle advantage, weight loss, higher athletic basic performance, or regular well-being. Tailoring electricity schooling starts offevolved offevolved with aligning bodily sports activities with particular aspirations.

Assessing Fitness Levels:

A critical step in customization is assessing modern-day-day health degrees. The chapter discusses diverse assessment techniques, from clean bodily sports to more advanced metrics, supporting humans gauge their power, flexibility, and endurance. Understanding baseline fitness informs the layout of a customized energy training program.

Adapting for Beginners:

For beginners, embarking on a power training journey may be intimidating. This segment offers insights into easing beginners into strength education, emphasizing proper form, grade by grade growing intensity, and incorporating foundational bodily video games. Tailoring for beginners fosters a exceptional and sustainable creation to electricity training.

Progressive Overload Principles:

Tailoring strength education includes making use of modern overload ideas. Exploring the concept of often developing resistance, quantity, or intensity, the chapter elucidates how this crucial precept stimulates chronic versions, selling sustained profits in energy tailored to person abilties.

Modifying for Advanced Fitness Levels:

Advanced health enthusiasts require tailor-made techniques to constantly mission their our our bodies. The phase delves into advanced electricity schooling techniques, which encompass periodization, diverse rep tiers, and incorporating superior bodily sports. Customization for superior stages ensures ongoing development and forestalls plateaus.

Addressing Health Considerations:

Individual health troubles play a pivotal function in customization. This element explores how elements at the facet of pre-current situations, accidents, or mobility limitations impact energy training. Tailoring wearing events to house fitness considerations ensures a secure and powerful strength education experience.

Incorporating Preferences and Enjoyment:

Sustainability in energy education is cautiously associated with leisure. The financial catastrophe discusses how incorporating selections, whether or not or now not thru desire of wearing occasions, workout surroundings, or education style, contributes to extended-time period adherence. Tailoring energy training to align with individual alternatives fosters a amazing and exciting health enjoy.

Balancing Frequency and Duration:

Tailoring power schooling includes finding the right balance between workout frequency and length. The segment offers insights into crafting a time table that aligns with individual time constraints, ensuring that strength education stays a possible and critical a part of one's ordinary.

Customization for Age-Related Factors:

As people age, energy schooling requirements evolve. This component addresses the way to tailor power schooling packages to address age-related elements inclusive of joint health, restoration time, and trendy fitness goals. Customization for particular age groups guarantees that electricity training remains beneficial and available in the course of the lifespan.

Individualizing Recovery Strategies:

Recognizing the individualized nature of restoration is crucial. The bankruptcy explores tailor-made recovery techniques, which includes nutrients, sleep, and lively restoration strategies. Customizing healing ensures that individuals optimize the blessings of electricity training whilst minimizing the risk of burnout or overtraining.

Personalized Recovery Protocols:

An essential factor of customization lies in tailoring nutrients to complement power schooling. This phase explores customized nutritional issues, which include caloric intake, macronutrient ratios, and hydration. Recognizing that character our our bodies reply in a one-of-a-type manner to nutritional strategies, this financial ruin guides readers in aligning vitamins with their unique dreams and desires.

Integrating Functional Movements:

Tailoring energy education consists of integrating useful actions that align with each day sports activities. This element highlights the importance of incorporating bodily sports that mimic real-existence motions, enhancing now not simplest power but also the realistic applicability of the training. Functional moves make a contribution to improved functionality in every day obligations, a key interest in customization.

Personalized Recovery Protocols:

Recovery is a specially individualized issue of electricity schooling. The bankruptcy delves into customized recuperation protocols, alongside aspect techniques for managing muscle pain, optimizing sleep styles, and incorporating active recovery techniques. Tailoring recovery acknowledges the suitable necessities of each character, selling sustained properly-being sooner or later of the education journey.

Psychological Considerations in Customization:

Beyond the physical realm, mental factors play a pivotal feature in customization. This segment explores how man or woman motivations, mind-set, and options impact the effectiveness of energy training. Tailoring techniques to align with mental elements ensures a exceptional and empowering experience, fostering prolonged-term adherence to energy education dreams.

Tracking Progress and Adjusting Plans:

A key issue of tailoring strength schooling consists of non-stop evaluation and adjustment. The financial ruin provides insights into effective techniques of monitoring improvement, whether or not or not or now not through wellknown common performance metrics, electricity gains, or subjective remarks. Understanding the way to evolve plans based on improvement guarantees that individuals live engaged and stimulated in their custom designed strength training adventure.

Empowering Self-Efficacy:

Customization is a powerful tool in enhancing self-efficacy—the perception in a single's capacity to accumulate preferred results. This detail explores how tailoring electricity education empowers human beings with the useful resource of manner of aligning bodily video games with non-public alternatives, competencies, and aspirations. Strengthening self-efficacy contributes to sustained determination and enthusiasm for the electricity education journey.

Building a Supportive Environment:

Creating a supportive environment is essential for personalisation achievement. The segment discusses the importance of social aid, whether or now not from pals, own family, or a health community. Tailoring electricity schooling to align with an person's social context fosters a enjoy of belonging and encouragement, reinforcing the willpower to fitness goals.

Case Studies in Customization:

To offer practical insights, this monetary disaster consists of case research illustrating success customization techniques. These actual-international examples display how people with diverse desires and competencies tailor-made their electricity schooling sports, showcasing the versatility and effectiveness of customization in accomplishing various fitness goals.

Chapter 4: Functional Movement Strategies for Daily Activities

In this monetary spoil, we delve into realistic and sensible motion techniques tailor-made to enhance your each day sports sports. The motive is to mix sporting sports activities seamlessly into your habitual, promoting now not only physical properly-being however moreover stepped forward efficiency and simplicity in performing regular duties.

Understanding Functional Movements:

Functional actions are those who mimic actual-existence sports and have interaction a couple of muscle organizations, promoting coordination and electricity. This segment introduces the concept of useful movements and their relevance to each day activities, laying the muse for the techniques that follow.

Morning Mobility Routine:

Start your day with a tough and speedy of mobility physical sports designed to wake up your body and prepare it for the day earlier. This ordinary consists of mild stretches, joint movements, and stability sporting events to promote flexibility and mobility, setting a amazing tone for the day.

Incorporating Functional Exercises into Household Chores:

Discover how normal chores can double as possibilities for practical sporting sports. From squats whilst loading the dishwasher to lunges on the same time as vacuuming, this section offers sensible recommendations on infusing your family duties with realistic actions.

Desk-positive Mobility Breaks:

For people with sedentary jobs, this aspect offers a chain of short mobility breaks to fight the results of prolonged sitting. Simple stretches, seated leg lifts, and shoulder rolls can be seamlessly blanketed into your art work recurring to beautify move and reduce stiffness.

Walking Techniques for Improved Functionality:

Walking is a essential each day interest, and optimizing your on foot approach can also have massive-ranging advantages. Explore pointers on posture, stride length, and arm movement to make your walks not first-rate fun but moreover conducive to common sensible health.

Staircase Workouts for Strength and Endurance:

If you have get right of entry to to stairs, they end up a treasured aid for realistic physical activities. Learn a manner to leverage staircases for physical games that target leg strength, cardiovascular fitness, and balance, reworking a commonplace characteristic right right into a health tool.

Functional Movements for Joint Health:

Maintaining joint fitness is important for each day mobility. This section introduces sensible movements mainly designed to sell joint flexibility and energy. Exercises concentrated on the hips, knees, and shoulders make a contribution to traditional joint nicely-being.

Dynamic Stretching Before Daily Activities:

Incorporating dynamic stretching into your pre-interest ordinary can decorate flexibility and decrease the hazard of injuries. This detail gives a set of dynamic stretches appropriate for severa every day sports activities, ensuring your frame is primed for movement.

Evening Relaxation Routine:

Wrap up your day with a chilled ordinary designed to sell rest and versatility. Gentle stretches, deep breathing sporting activities, and mindfulness strategies make a contribution to winding down every bodily and mentally.

Expanding on Daily Activity Integration:

Building upon the concept of incorporating useful moves into every day sports activities, this segment provides extra examples and modern thoughts. Whether it's miles turning family chores into full-frame physical games or finding opportunities for useful moves in some unspecified time within the future of entertainment sports activities activities, the goal is to make workout seamlessly woven into the material of your daily existence.

Seated Functional Exercises for Office Settings:

For those spending prolonged hours in an office placing, this part introduces a sequence of seated practical sporting occasions. These wearing sports activities goal middle power, posture, and flexibility, addressing the demanding situations of table-high quality workouts and promoting an lively technique to place of work-based totally fitness.

Functional Movement Breaks:

Recognizing the significance of taking breaks at a few level inside the day, this segment introduces the idea of sensible motion breaks. Short, focused bursts of motion can reenergize every frame and thoughts. From brief stretches to mini-exercise exercises, the ones breaks purpose to beautify productivity and nicely-being.

Adapting Functional Movements for Varied Fitness Levels:

Understanding that humans have awesome fitness tiers, this element explores the way to adapt sensible moves to fit varying abilties. Whether you're a amateur or have advanced fitness, the sporting sports activities furnished can be tailor-made to satisfy your contemporary fitness degree, making sure inclusivity and accessibility.

Functional Movements for Enhanced Posture:

Good posture is crucial to every day sports sports and regular properly-being. This segment focuses on useful actions that target center electricity and postural muscle mass. By incorporating these physical video games into your everyday, you can artwork within the path of improving posture, decreasing ache, and improving frame interest.

Integrating Functional Movements into Recreation:

Leisure sports activities present opportunities for useful moves. Whether you enjoy gardening, gambling sports activities, or venture amusement pastimes, this difficulty explores the manner to infuse the ones sports activities with beneficial sports. This holistic method guarantees that your amusement time contributes to each leisure and bodily health.

Addressing Common Daily Movement Challenges:

This section addresses common stressful conditions people face of their daily movements. From addressing stiffness within the morning to combating fatigue inside the afternoon, sensible solutions and bodily sports are supplied to triumph over the ones worrying conditions and hold a constant level of strength and energy for the duration of the day.

Functional Movement Apps and Resources:

Explore the vicinity of practical movement apps and sources designed to guide and encourage your each day exercising ordinary. From guided exercising apps to movement tracking tools, this element introduces technological aids that may enhance your engagement with practical bodily video games.

Measuring Progress in Daily Functional Fitness:

Understanding the impact of realistic motion techniques requires tracking development. This segment gives insights into the way to measure enhancements in power, flexibility, and often occurring useful health. Establishing benchmarks and celebrating small victories make a contribution to the ongoing fulfillment of your every day beneficial fitness adventure.

Encouraging Consistency through Habit Formation:

Consistency is fundamental in reaping the blessings of functional motion techniques. This element explores the technological expertise of dependancy formation and offers sensible pointers for incorporating these physical games into your recurring typically. By establishing conduct, you make certain that useful movements come to be an critical a part of your every day existence.

4.1: Integrating Functional Movements into Everyday Life

In this phase, we delve into the realistic components of seamlessly integrating sensible moves into your everyday life. By making physical video

video games an inherent part of your habitual, you now not simplest decorate physical fitness however moreover domesticate a conscious method to motion inside the context of your every day activities.

Functional Movements in Daily Chores:

Explore how recurring household chores may be converted into sensible physical video games. From squatting on the equal time as choosing up groceries to incorporating lunges at the identical time as making the bed, this element gives insights into infusing practical actions into your daily chores, turning mundane responsibilities into opportunities for bodily engagement.

Walking with Purpose:

Walking is a crucial every day interest, and this section emphasizes walking with motive. Whether it's miles specializing in maintaining right posture, incorporating brisk intervals, or attractive your fingers for a complete-frame workout, find out how to show your every day walk into a practical exercising that contributes on your not unusual properly-being.

Active Commuting Strategies:

For folks that pass backward and forward often, this element explores methods to make your journey more lively. From incorporating standing stretches on public delivery to selecting stairs over escalators, the ones techniques make sure that your travel becomes an possibility for moderate exercise, selling waft and power.

Desk-certain Functional Movements:

Address the challenges of sedentary place of business art work thru introducing beneficial actions that can be seamlessly integrated into your workday. Simple physical video games like seated leg lifts, table push-ups, and shoulder rolls are provided to fight the horrible effects of prolonged sitting and sell a greater lively art work environment.

Functional Breaks During Screen Time:

Screen time regularly dominates our every day wearing sports, and this segment indicates incorporating sensible breaks into prolonged intervals of sitting. Quick stretches, eye bodily sports, and seated twists are introduced to counteract the sedentary nature of show-related sports activities sports, fostering motion and reducing stiffness.

Functional Movements in Social Settings:

Discover how social gatherings and outings can end up possibilities for useful moves. Whether it's far incorporating status stretches at some stage in a conversation or choosing activities that contain physical engagement, this part encourages a social environment that allows both connection and fitness.

Family Fitness Routines:

For families, growing health sporting activities together enhances each bodily fitness and bonding. This phase gives thoughts for family-notable practical sports that cater to one-of-a-type age agencies. From outside video video games to group sports activities, fostering a manner of life of family health turns into an exciting and shared enjoy.

Shopping as a Functional Exercise:

Turn your purchasing trips into practical carrying occasions by way of the use of incorporating functional movements. This detail indicates techniques to interact your muscle corporations at the same time as navigating the aisles, wearing baggage, and loading your groceries. By making purchasing for an lively enjoy, you're making contributions for your common health with out dedicating particular exercising time.

Mindful Movement Practices:

Integrate mindfulness into your day by day actions by using adopting conscious movement practices. This phase explores the advantages of being observed in every motion, emphasizing the thoughts-body connection. By incorporating mindfulness, you now not wonderful decorate the effectiveness of your beneficial carrying sports activities but moreover cultivate a experience of tranquility.

Functional Movements in Outdoor Activities:

Explore how outdoor sports can be enriched with practical movements. Whether it's far hiking, gardening, or playing recreational sports, this section suggests incorporating useful sporting occasions that align with the natural waft of those activities. By making the most of the outside environment, you enhance each your health and reference to nature.

Functional Movements in Cooking and Meal Prep:

The kitchen becomes a dynamic area for purposeful actions as this factor introduces sports that can be seamlessly included into cooking and meal steering. From repute stability wearing occasions on the same time as stirring to incorporating squats even as ready, the ones movements contribute for your day by day hobby ranges.

Stairs as a Functional Exercise Tool:

If you've got stairs for your daily surroundings, this phase explores leveraging them as a precious tool for useful exercising. Stair mountain climbing engages multiple muscle corporations and complements cardiovascular health. Learn top notch stair carrying activities and techniques for making stair use a beneficial part of your each day everyday.

Functional Movements for Enhanced Posture at Work:

For those spending prolonged hours at a table, preserving proper posture is vital. This detail introduces beneficial movements specifically geared closer to enhancing posture in some unspecified time in the future of labor hours. From seated stretches to midday posture resets, the ones wearing events counteract the effects of extended sitting on posture and musculoskeletal fitness.

Functional Movements During Leisure Screen Time:

Even in the course of leisure screen time, practical actions can be protected to offset sedentary behavior. This segment shows bodily games which incorporates seated leg extensions or neck stretches while looking TV or the use of digital devices. By incorporating motion into relaxation time, you sell a balance between display display display screen-based totally enjoyment and bodily hobby.

Functional Movements for Improved Sleep:

Explore how incorporating unique beneficial moves into your pre-sleep ordinary can make contributions to higher sleep first rate. Gentle stretches, relaxation carrying activities, and mindful respiratory techniques are brought to create a bedtime ritual that now not simplest relaxes the frame however moreover enhances sizable sleep hygiene.

Multi-tasking with Functional Movements:

Discover the art work of multi-tasking with the beneficial aid of incorporating functional movements into sports activities that normally incorporate most effective one attention. Whether it's running towards balance physical video games even as brushing your enamel or doing calf will boom whilst watching for the kettle to boil, this phase encourages performance in making the maximum of it sluggish.

Functional Movements for Stress Reduction:

Recognizing the impact of pressure on popular well-being, this element introduces practical actions that especially goal stress bargain. Exercises in conjunction with deep breathing, slight stretches, and aware movements make a contribution to developing moments of calm inner your worrying agenda.

Daily Movement Journaling:

Consider keeping a every day movement journal to tune your development and mirror at the combination of beneficial actions into your regular life. This phase affords guidance on retaining a smooth magazine that lets in you live responsible, set goals, and feature a first-rate time the successes to your journey within the route of a greater energetic way of life.

Creating a Personalized Daily Movement Plan:

Tailor realistic moves for your particular every day schedule through the usage of growing a custom designed motion plan. This aspect gives realistic recommendations on assessing your daily ordinary, figuring out opportunities for motion, and growing a plan that aligns together together with your desires and possibilities.

four.2: Enhancing Daily Activities through Purposeful Exercises

This phase specializes in the intentional enhancement of each day sports through practical sporting sports. By infusing your habitual with centered movements, you not simplest make bigger the overall overall performance of everyday obligations but additionally make contributions for your everyday bodily well-being.

Functional Movements in Household Chores:

Explore how useful physical activities can growth the impact of family chores. From incorporating squats at the same time as loading the dishwasher to appearing lunges whilst vacuuming, this detail gives practical examples of procedures every day sports can grow to be opportunities for muscle engagement and conditioning.

Efficient Movement Patterns:

Discover the idea of green movement patterns and the manner they're able to streamline every day duties. This section emphasizes optimizing body mechanics in the route of sports activities like lifting, accomplishing, and sporting to lessen the danger of stress or harm. Learn how easy modifications in motion can extensively decorate the effectiveness of day by day moves.

Balance and Stability Exercises:

Integrate stability and balance sports activities sports into daily sports activities to enhance common coordination. From repute on one leg whilst brushing your tooth to incorporating stability demanding conditions on the same time as achieving for devices, this detail offers sporting sports that improve proprioception and assist better manage of movement.

Postural Awareness in Daily Tasks:

Develop postural reputation in some unspecified time in the future of everyday sports activities activities to sell spinal health and muscle engagement. This segment explores maintaining a independent spine even as sitting, fame, and bending to prevent undue stress at the lower lower back. By incorporating postural principles, you make a contribution to prolonged-time period musculoskeletal nicely-being.

Functional Movements in Work Tasks:

Apply sensible physical video games to enhance art work-related obligations. Whether it's miles incorporating seated leg lifts in the path of table paintings or integrating fame stretches into quick breaks, this element gives techniques for infusing movement into the workday. By optimizing movement at artwork, you assist physical fitness and productivity.

Efficient Movement During Commuting:

Explore strategies to make commuting extra than just a method of transportation. This section shows realistic wearing occasions like isometric contractions all through transit or enticing your center at the identical time as the usage of. By making your tour an active a part of your day, you are making contributions to average every day movement goals.

Purposeful Movements While Waiting:

Transform moments of ready into possibilities for practical sports activities sports. Whether it's far calf will increase on the identical time as popularity in line or seated stretches for the duration of a wait, this thing encourages turning idle time into lively moments. Learn a manner to make the most of these intervals to build up useful movement all through the day.

Joint Mobility Exercises for Daily Flexibility:

Incorporate joint mobility bodily activities into each day exercise workouts to beautify flexibility. From mild neck rotations to ankle circles, this section presents sporting activities that lubricate joints and sell standard mobility. By prioritizing joint health, you make sure a greater form of motion in each day sports activities sports.

Functional Movements in Leisure Activities:

Enhance amusement time with realistic sporting events that complement leisure sports activities. Whether it's miles integrating stretches into reading time or acting mild physical video video games in the course of display-based totally definitely amusement, this issue shows techniques to infuse movement into moments of rest.

Mindful Eating Practices:

Explore the concept of aware consuming as a useful workout. This section encourages listening to frame cues, taking breaks amongst bites, and incorporating diffused moves like seated twists. By fostering popularity at some stage in meals, you not first-rate assist digestion however additionally introduce useful actions.

Functional Movements in Social Gatherings:

Turn social gatherings into opportunities for useful bodily games. This element suggests incorporating popularity stretches, gentle moves, or maybe business enterprise sports activities at some point of social sports. By developing an environment that encourages each connection and motion, you are making a contribution to a holistic approach to fitness.

Functional Movements for Improved Sleep:

Discover how incorporating unique useful movements into your pre-sleep habitual can contribute to higher sleep tremendous. Gentle stretches, relaxation sporting sports activities, and conscious respiratory strategies are brought to create a bedtime ritual that now not best relaxes the frame but moreover complements typical sleep hygiene.

Multi-tasking with Functional Movements:

Explore the art of multi-tasking thru incorporating sensible movements into sports that normally consist of most effective one cognizance. Whether it's miles working inside the course of balance bodily video games while brushing your enamel or doing calf will increase on the identical time as watching for the kettle to boil, this phase encourages overall performance in making the most of it sluggish.

Functional Movements for Stress Reduction:

Recognizing the impact of strain on desired nicely-being, this thing introduces sensible actions that mainly reason strain discount. Exercises together with deep breathing, mild stretches, and mindful movements make a contribution to developing moments of calm internal your demanding schedule.

Daily Movement Journaling:

Consider maintaining a each day motion mag to music your improvement and replicate at the combination of sensible movements into your normal existence. This section offers steerage on retaining a smooth mag that lets in you live responsible, set dreams, and feature a laugh the successes to your adventure within the course of a greater lively way of lifestyles.

Creating a Personalized Daily Movement Plan:

Tailor practical movements on your unique each day schedule through way of growing a customized motion plan. This thing gives sensible tips on assessing your each day regular, figuring out possibilities for movement, and developing a plan that aligns along facet your goals and alternatives.

Chapter 5: The Scale Is Not a Useful Tool for Measuring Results

Challenge the conventional method to measuring health development thru the usage of thinking the effectiveness of the scale. This bankruptcy delves into the policies of using weight due to the fact the primary metric for achievement and advocates for a more holistic and useful mindset on fitness and fitness.

Understanding the Scale's Limitations:

Explore the pitfalls of depending mostly on weight as a measure of health. This segment discusses how factors like water retention, muscle advantage, and body composition can have an impact at the numbers on the size, regularly imparting an incomplete and deceptive image of 1's not unusual fitness and well-being.

Rethinking Traditional Measurement Metrics:

Encourage readers to shift their attention from weight-centric metrics to extra great symptoms and signs and symptoms of development. This issue introduces opportunity measurements which includes frame composition evaluation, power levels, and realistic improvements as greater correct reflections of someone's fitness journey.

Emphasizing Functional Progress Over Scale Numbers:

Highlight the importance of realistic development as a actual degree of fitness achievement. This segment emphasizes how improvements in strength, flexibility, persistence, and common functionality offer a more complete and reliable gauge of 1's well-being in comparison to arbitrary numbers on a scale.

Functional Fitness Assessments:

Introduce useful health checks as precious gear for monitoring development. This component discusses tests that diploma mobility, balance, and agility, providing a more insightful evaluation of an man or woman's fitness journey beyond what conventional scales can provide.

Case Studies:

Illustrate the shortcomings of depending completely on weight via real-life case studies. Share memories of individuals who skilled large beneficial enhancements without massive weight reduction, demonstrating the importance of looking beyond the size for a more correct assessment.

Importance of Non-Scale Victories:

Celebrate non-scale victories as vital milestones inside the health adventure. This segment explores achievements which incorporates progressed sleep, elevated strength levels, stronger temper, and a notable thoughts-set as precious markers of success that pass past the numeric popularity of traditional weight measurements.

Embracing a Mindful Approach:

Advocate for a conscious technique to fitness and fitness. This issue encourages readers to tune into their our our bodies, listen to how they revel in, and understand the super modifications happening internally, fostering a more sustainable and holistic mind-set within the course of well-being.

Setting Meaningful Goals:

Guide readers in placing goals that boom beyond the dimensions. This section permits people find out personal, beneficial, and typical overall performance-based totally goals, imparting a roadmap for a fulfilling and motive-driven fitness adventure.

Tracking Functional Progress:

Offer sensible recommendation on the manner to track realistic development correctly. Whether thru journaling, incorporating health apps, or utilizing health checks, this element equips readers with equipment to screen upgrades that align with their precise fitness desires.

Understanding Body Composition:

Dive deeper into the concept of frame composition and its importance in assessing fitness. This phase explains how records the distribution of muscle, fat, and other tissues gives a extra nuanced mind-set on physical fitness in assessment to relying absolutely on standard body weight.

Impact of Muscle Gain:

Explore the high-quality impact of muscle advantage on ordinary health. This detail breaks down the false impression that weight advantage continuously equals fats gain, highlighting how constructing muscle can contribute to a leaner and more healthy frame. Encourage readers to understand the characteristic of muscle in beneficial health.

Debunking Weight Loss Myths:

Address commonplace weight reduction myths that perpetuate misconceptions about health and health. This phase interests to debunk notions which incorporates speedy weight loss equating to advanced health, emphasizing the significance of sustainable and realistic progress over brief fixes.

Functional Fitness Success Stories:

Share inspiring success stories of individuals who performed extraordinary useful health improvements with out outstanding weight reduction. These narratives function effective examples of methods focusing on purposeful desires can purpose transformative changes in widespread nicely-being.

Educating on Metabolic Health:

Educate readers on the connection amongst weight, metabolism, and everyday fitness. Discuss how metabolic fitness, inspired by using approach of factors beyond weight, plays a crucial function in identifying one's properly-being. This phase empowers people to prioritize metabolic fitness over arbitrary weight dreams.

Mind-Body Connection:

Explore the mind-body connection and its impact on famous health. This detail delves into how pressure, highbrow well-being, and emotional fitness can have an effect on physical fitness and, consequently, the effectiveness of health trips. Encourage a holistic technique to nicely-being.

Functional Fitness Challenges:

Present demanding situations that focus on useful fitness rather than weight loss. This segment introduces readers to sensible disturbing conditions that emphasize improvements in energy, flexibility, and endurance. These traumatic conditions feature motivational equipment for the ones seeking out a extra practical and gratifying fitness adventure.

Integrating Functional Metrics:

Guide readers on integrating useful metrics into their health assessments. Whether it is monitoring the capability to perform each day sports with greater ease or measuring upgrades in precise sports activities, this element offers tangible techniques to shift the focal point from the dimensions to substantial realistic signs and symptoms.

Community Support and Accountability:

Highlight the importance of community help in fostering a thoughts-set shift away from the scale. Discuss how duty companions, health communities, or guide networks can make contributions to a extraordinary environment that encourages useful development and celebrates diverse definitions of success.

Building a Resilient Mindset:

Empower readers with strategies to construct a resilient mindset in their health journeys. This phase gives system for overcoming setbacks, embracing screw ups as gaining knowledge of opportunities, and cultivating a extremely good outlook that is going beyond the numbers on a scale

5.1: Rethinking Traditional Measurement Metrics

Challenge the set up norms in fitness assessment through using thinking the effectiveness of conventional length metrics. This chapter delves into the rules of the usage of weight due to the fact the number one metric for achievement and advocates for a greater holistic and functional attitude on health and fitness improvement.

Shortcomings of Traditional Metrics:

Discuss the restrictions of traditional metrics along side frame weight, BMI, and calorie counting. Explore how the ones metrics regularly fail to provide a whole facts of an character's common health and health degree, neglecting important factors like body composition, muscle tissues, and useful talents.

Body Composition as a Key Indicator:

Highlight the significance of body composition as a greater accurate indicator of health. Explain how facts the ratio of muscle to fats gives valuable insights into metabolic fitness, physical common performance, and usual well-being. Encourage readers to prioritize frame composition exams over simplistic weight-targeted metrics.

Functional Fitness Metrics:

Introduce the concept of practical health metrics that go beyond the traditional measurements. Discuss the importance of assessing energy, flexibility, agility, and endurance as essential components of a holistic health evaluation. Emphasize how the ones metrics align extra intently with the desires of useful schooling.

Tailoring Metrics to Individual Goals:

Advocate for a customized method to fitness metrics primarily based totally on man or woman desires. This phase courses readers in deciding on metrics that align with their unique aspirations, whether or now not it is improving athletic average standard overall performance, enhancing day by day sports activities, or accomplishing particular functional milestones.

Mindful Eating and Intuitive Metrics:

Explore the characteristic of conscious consuming and intuitive metrics in fostering a extra wholesome relationship with food. Discuss how listening to hunger cues, nourishing the frame with nutrient-dense substances, and cultivating conscious eating behavior can make a contribution to commonplace properly-being, going beyond calorie-centric measurements.

Emotional and Mental Health Metrics:

Acknowledge the effect of emotional and intellectual fitness on regular properly-being. Introduce the concept of incorporating emotional intelligence, pressure management, and intellectual health checks as important metrics inside the fitness adventure. Highlight the interconnectedness of highbrow and bodily fitness.

Holistic Wellness Metrics:

Promote a holistic method to nicely being thru thinking about a broader spectrum of metrics. Discuss the inclusion of sleep first-class, energy levels, temper, and usual existence delight as valuable indicators of a properly-rounded and thriving way of existence. Encourage readers to view health as a multidimensional concept.

Progress Journals and Tracking:

Encourage using development journals for monitoring a severa set of metrics. Provide steering on growing custom designed journals that embody physical, emotional, and life-style metrics. Emphasize the charge of mirrored picture and self-attention in the adventure inside the path of top-super health.

Educational Resources for Metric Understanding:

Provide hints for educational resources that empower human beings to apprehend and interpret severa health metrics. This thing equips readers with the know-how had to make knowledgeable choices approximately their health and fitness, fostering a experience of autonomy and self-empowerment.

Exploring Holistic Wellness Metrics:

Delve deeper into the idea of holistic well-being metrics, emphasizing the interconnectedness of various factors of well-being. Discuss how metrics which includes sleep great, strain degrees, emotional stability, and life satisfaction contribute to a extra entire data of an individual's traditional fitness. Encourage readers to boom their mind-set beyond bodily metrics by myself.

Customizing Metrics for Personal Goals:

Guide readers in tailoring metrics to align with their specific fitness and fitness targets. Whether aiming for weight reduction, muscle benefit, stepped forward athletic average standard performance, or progressed every day functionality, this segment gives practical advice on choosing metrics that proper away correlate with character goals.

Utilizing Technology for Metric Tracking:

Introduce the location of technology in modern-day-day metric tracking. Discuss the benefits of fitness apps, wearables, and clever gadgets that allow people to show various factors of their health and fitness journey. Emphasize how the ones equipment can enhance recognition, motivation, and adherence to custom designed metrics.

The Role of Professional Guidance:

Highlight the importance of seeking out professional steering in understanding and interpreting fitness metrics. Encourage readers to looking for advice from health specialists, nutritionists, and healthcare companies to get maintain of personalized insights into their particular metrics and to ensure a strong and effective health journey.

Empowering Mindful Eating:

Expand at the concept of conscious ingesting as a metric for dietary nicely-being. Provide sensible recommendations on developing conscious ingesting behavior, recognizing starvation and fullness cues, and fostering a effective dating with food. Showcase how mindfulness in consuming can contribute to stepped forward dietary alternatives and average health.

Incorporating Lifestyle Metrics:

Explore the inclusion of way of life metrics that pass beyond conventional fitness assessments. Discuss how factors like each day movement, sedentary behavior, and amusement sports activities make contributions to ordinary health. Guide readers in spotting and optimizing way of existence metrics for a greater holistic technique to properly-being.

Measuring Emotional Resilience:

Discuss the vicinity of emotional resilience as a metric for mental well-being. Explore how humans can check their functionality to deal with strain, setbacks, and demanding situations. Provide realistic techniques for enhancing emotional resilience, emphasizing its significance in maintaining traditional health and fitness.

Creating a Personalized Metric Toolkit:

Empower readers to create their custom designed metric toolkit.

Offer a whole manual on deciding on, tracking, and interpreting metrics that align with character values and aspirations. Encourage the mixture of severa metrics to color a more correct and personalised photo of health and health.

Promoting a Growth Mindset:

Encourage the adoption of a boom thoughts-set at the same time as coming near metrics. Emphasize that metrics are equipment for studying and development in place of strict measures of achievement or failure. Foster a amazing and adaptive mindset that permits people to encompass stressful conditions, studies from critiques, and constantly evolve on their health adventure.

5.2: Emphasizing Functional Progress Over Scale Numbers

Shift the point of interest from conventional scale numbers to the significance of practical improvement inside the health adventure. This chapter advocates for a holistic method that prioritizes improvements in beneficial talents over simplistic weight-oriented metrics.

Challenges with Scale Numbers:

Discuss the restrictions of relying totally on scale numbers for gauging health success. Address the commonplace pitfalls, alongside aspect overlooking muscle advantage, neglecting frame composition adjustments, and fostering an horrible fixation on weight loss. Highlight how scale numbers regularly fail to seize the broader spectrum of enhancements.

Defining Functional Progress:

Introduce the idea of beneficial improvement, emphasizing

improvements in energy, flexibility, mobility, and regular functionality. Illustrate how the ones factors make a contribution to stepped forward each day existence, extra athletic typical normal overall performance, and a greater resilient and succesful frame. Encourage readers to redefine their definition of fulfillment inside the health adventure.

Functional Fitness Benchmarks:

Present some of useful fitness benchmarks that increase past weight-associated dreams. Discuss how conducting milestones like reading unique sports activities, growing stamina, or improving joint mobility can feature powerful signs of progress. Showcase the power of sensible benchmarks in assessing average health.

Measuring Strength and Endurance:

Explore the significance of measuring power and staying strength as key additives of beneficial improvement. Provide insights into how improvements in lifting heavier weights, appearing greater repetitions, or keeping physical sports for longer intervals replicate improvements in muscular and cardiovascular health.

Assessing Flexibility and Mobility:

Highlight the placement of flexibility and mobility checks in monitoring beneficial improvement. Discuss how expanded form of movement, advanced joint flexibility, and extra tremendous mobility make contributions to better motion styles, reduced damage risk, and common practical properly-being.

Functional Movement Patterns:

Discuss the significance of learning beneficial motion styles as a degree of development. Explore how wearing occasions that mimic real-life moves, inclusive of squats, lunges, and twists, can translate into advanced common performance in each day activities. Emphasize the connection among practical moves and greater suited wonderful of existence.

Adapting Workouts for Functional Gains:

Provide realistic advice on adapting exercising exercises to reputation on useful earnings. Discuss the incorporation of compound wearing activities, entire-frame moves, and sundry exercising modalities that prioritize beneficial fitness. Guide readers in designing sporting activities that align with their individual realistic goals.

The Role of Consistency:

Emphasize the feature of consistency in sporting out sensible improvement.

Discuss how everyday, sustainable efforts contribute to lengthy-term enhancements in practical competencies. Encourage readers to embody the adventure and feature an first-rate time incremental useful profits as markers of fulfillment.

Celebrating Non-Scale Victories:

Encourage readers to have an notable time non-scale victories as powerful motivators. Explore the emotional and intellectual effect of acknowledging and appreciating improvements in purposeful capabilities. Foster a extremely good thoughts-set that acknowledges the price of the entire health journey, past numerical measurements.

Progress Tracking Beyond Weight:

Encourage readers to diversify their technique to development monitoring beyond weight-associated metrics. Discuss the relevance of body measurements, adjustments in garb wholesome, and visual improvement pics as alternative strategies to degree the effect of health efforts. Highlight how these signs and symptoms offer a more entire view of bodily transformation.

Holistic Wellness Metrics:

Integrate the concept of holistic well being metrics into the talk, emphasizing how improvements in sleep remarkable, stress manipulate, and number one nicely-being make a contribution to practical development. Illustrate the interconnectedness of severa life-style factors and their effect on each physical and highbrow fitness.

Functional Progress in Daily Activities:

Explore how beneficial improvement right now interprets into advanced performance in every day activities. Discuss actual-life examples of human beings who've expert higher ease in obligations which incorporates lifting groceries, mountain climbing stairs, or playing with youngsters because of their realistic fitness improvements. Reinforce the idea that proper fulfillment extends past the fitness center.

Adaptive Exercise Modifications:

Provide guidance on adaptive exercising changes that accommodate person needs and stressful conditions.

Discuss how people with amazing fitness degrees, frame kinds, or health situations can tailor their physical games to emphasise purposeful improvement. Encourage inclusivity in fitness with the useful aid of showcasing numerous strategies to practical training.

Functional Progress Assessments:

Introduce numerous checks for monitoring useful development. Discuss the usage of fitness assessments, movement screenings, and sensible evaluations to quantify enhancements particularly regions. Illustrate how the ones checks can function benchmarks for placing and accomplishing useful fitness dreams.

The Mind-Body Connection:

Explore the thoughts-body connection in the context of beneficial development. Discuss how a first-rate thoughts-set, intellectual resilience, and emotional nicely-being make contributions to average functional health. Emphasize that a holistic approach to health includes nurturing each physical and highbrow elements.

Educational Resources for Functional Fitness:

Provide guidelines for educational assets that empower human beings to recognize the requirements of practical fitness. Suggest books, articles, and on-line systems that provide insights into the technology and alertness of sensible training. Equip readers with the understanding needed to make knowledgeable alternatives about their health journey.

Community Support and Accountability:

Highlight the characteristic of network help and obligation in fostering sensible improvement. Discuss the advantages of turning into a member of health groups, taking element in organisation physical games, or seeking out steering from health specialists. Illustrate how a supportive environment can enhance motivation and adherence to purposeful health desires.

Overcoming Setbacks and Challenges:

Acknowledge that setbacks and stressful conditions are inherent in any health adventure. Provide techniques for overcoming limitations and staying resilient in the pursuit of realistic improvement. Share stories of individuals who have navigated setbacks and emerged more potent, reinforcing the concept that resilience is a vital element of the adventure

Chapter 6: Create Your Personal Fitness Journey

Embarking on a private health journey is a transformative and empowering desire. This monetary catastrophe is your guide to crafting a health plan that resonates together together with your desires, options, and manner of lifestyles. It's now not pretty a whole lot exercise; it's far a holistic approach to improving your everyday nicely-being. Let's delve deeper into the key factors if you want to shape your unique fitness adventure.

Setting Personalized Fitness Goals:

1. Define Your Objectives:

Begin through truely defining your fitness goals. Whether it is weight loss, muscle advantage, progressed staying electricity, or everyday properly-being, knowledge your specific goals paperwork the foundation of your custom designed health adventure.

2. SMART Goals:

Dive into the idea of SMART goals— Specific, Measurable, Achievable, Relevant, and Time-positive. Learn the manner to formulate dreams which may be practical, trackable, and tailored for your specific aspirations.

Designing a Sustainable Fitness Plan:

1. Fitness Preferences:

Explore diverse varieties of sporting occasions and sports to find out what resonates collectively along with your options. Whether it is strength education, aerobic, yoga, or a aggregate, a sustainable plan aligns with personal amusement.

2. Balancing Workouts:

Emphasize the significance of a balanced exercise regular. Include components for cardiovascular fitness, energy building, flexibility, and relaxation. A well-rounded technique addresses one-of-a-kind components of health and reduces monotony.

3. Progressive Overload:

Understand the principle of cutting-edge overload—step by step developing intensity to stimulate chronic version. Design exercise plans that challenge you with out risking damage.

4. Consistency and Variety:

Stress the fee of consistency even as incorporating variety. Maintain everyday exercising schedules on the identical time as exploring numerous sports activities to prevent boredom and keep motivation excessive.

five. Adaptability:

Acknowledge that lifestyles is dynamic, and fitness plans should be adaptable. Adjust your exercise exercises based totally totally on converting occasions, ensuring lengthy-term sustainability.

Balancing Nutrition and Exercise:

1. Nutritional Goals:

Discuss the synergy among nutrients and exercising. Guide you in placing nutritional desires that supplement your health goals, whether or now not it's weight control, muscle building, or typical health.

2. Hydration:

Highlight the importance of hydration in helping bodily interest. Provide sensible guidelines for keeping properly enough water consumption at some point of the day and sooner or later of workout sporting events.

three. Nutrient-Rich Choices:

Encourage a focal point on nutrient-dense meals that gas your frame for best performance. Discuss the importance of a well-balanced weight loss program wealthy in proteins, carbohydrates, fat, nutrients, and minerals.

Prioritizing Recovery:

1. Sleep and Rest:

Highlight the region of sleep and rest inside the recuperation tool. Discuss the effect of super sleep on normal well-being and muscle restoration. Provide strategies for reinforcing sleep hygiene.

2. Active Recovery:

Introduce the idea of active restoration, incorporating moderate sporting events, stretching, or sports sports like yoga on relaxation days. Emphasize that recovery is an crucial part of health improvement.

Building a Support System:

1. Accountability Partners:

Encourage you to enlist assist from buddies, family, or exercising buddies. Discuss the blessings of duty companions in staying endorsed and committed to fitness goals.

2. Online Communities:

Explore the location of online health companies and social media companies. Discuss how sharing reports, looking for recommendation, and celebrating achievements with like-minded humans can enhance motivation.

Reflection and Adaptation:

1. Regular Reflection:

Stress the significance of ordinary self-mirrored image at the fitness journey. Assess your development, have a good time achievements, and grow to be aware of regions for improvement.

2. Adapting Goals:

Discuss the opportunity of adapting fitness desires primarily based on changing instances, achievements, or evolving aspirations. Flexibility in purpose-placing contributes to sustained motivation.

As you navigate your personal health journey, hold in thoughts that it is a dynamic and ongoing method. Embrace the uniqueness of your route, live adaptable, and have fun the incredible changes going on on your lifestyles. Your willpower to health and nicely-being is a lifelong funding, and each breakthrough is a victory. Best of success on your journey!

6.1: Setting Personalized Fitness Goals

Setting personalized health goals is the cornerstone of a a fulfillment and enjoyable fitness adventure. In this segment, we are going to delve into the method of defining targets which might be particular to you, presenting direction and motive on your endeavors. Let's embark on step one closer to a more healthy and happier you.

1. Define Your Objectives:

The journey begins with a easy information of what you want to gain. Whether it's far weight loss, muscle advantage, more desirable staying energy, or fundamental well-being, outline your desires with clarity. Take the time to reflect on what definitely subjects to you.

2. SMART Goals:

Introduce the SMART requirements— Specific, Measurable, Achievable, Relevant, and Time-certain. Apply those requirements in your health goals. For example, in vicinity of a vague cause like "shed pounds," make it specific, measurable, viable internal a fixed time frame, and relevant for your vast nicely-being.

3. Long-Term and Short-Term Goals:

Distinguish amongst prolonged-time period and brief-time period desires. Long-term dreams provide a broader mind-set, at the identical time as quick-term goals damage down the adventure into practicable steps. This method allows you to have a great time achievements along the way and live stimulated.

4. Consider Your Lifestyle:

Tailor your fitness goals to your way of existence. Recognize the wishes of your day by day existence, paintings, and private commitments. Setting sensible goals that align together along with your agenda will boom the probability of adherence.

5. Personal Values and Motivation:

Align your fitness dreams at the side of your non-public values and motivations. Understand why the ones desires are important to you. Whether it's far stepped forward fitness on your own family, multiplied power for art work, or a non-public fulfillment, connecting your dreams for your values enhances their significance.

6. Account for Variety:

Embrace variety to your health dreams. Include fantastic dimensions which incorporates cardiovascular fitness, electricity training, flexibility, and mental well-being. A well-rounded technique ensures whole fitness and stops monotony.

7. Gradual Progression:

Plan for gradual progression. Avoid putting overly formidable goals which can bring about burnout or harm. Progress at a tempo that worrying conditions you without overwhelming your modern-day health level.

eight. Adaptability:

Acknowledge that situations trade. Your goals must be adaptable to life's fluctuations. Be organized to adjust your goals based on evolving priorities, surprising stressful situations, or new opportunities.

Setting customized health desires is a dynamic machine that requires introspection, making plans, and flexibility. As you define your targets, bear in mind that they will be uniquely yours, designed to enhance your properly-being and align on the side of your aspirations. Embrace this step with enthusiasm, and allow your goals be a supply of notion for your adventure to a extra healthy and happier life-style.

6.2: Designing a Sustainable Fitness Plan for Long-Term Success

Congratulations on defining your custom designed fitness desires! Now, permit's transition to the subsequent important step—designing a sustainable fitness plan. This segment will guide you in crafting a holistic technique that ensures lengthy-time period fulfillment, incorporating balance, adaptability, and entertainment.

1. Fitness Preferences:

Explore diverse varieties of bodily sports to end up privy to what resonates with you. Whether it's miles power training, cardio, yoga, or a combination, a sustainable plan aligns with sports you virtually enjoy. This guarantees consistency and will increase the hazard of adherence.

2. Balancing Workouts:

Emphasize the importance of a balanced exercising regular. Incorporate additives for cardiovascular health, power building, flexibility, and rest. A well-rounded technique addresses one-of-a-type components of fitness, reducing the threat of overtraining and monotony.

three. Progressive Overload:

Introduce the precept of innovative overload. Gradually growth the depth of your exercising exercises to stimulate persistent version. This no longer most effective enhances physical general overall performance but additionally prevents plateaus and continues your health adventure dynamic.

four. Consistency and Variety:

Stress the fee of consistency whilst incorporating variety. Maintain regular exercising schedules at the same time as exploring numerous sports activities to prevent boredom and maintain motivation immoderate. Consistency builds conduct, and variety maintains your health routine thrilling.

five. Adaptability:

Acknowledge that lifestyles is dynamic, and fitness plans need to be adaptable. Encourage the capability to alter your exercises based totally on changing instances, making sure prolonged-time period sustainability. Adaptability is crucial to overcoming disturbing conditions and staying dedicated.

Balancing Nutrition and Exercise:

6. Nutritional Goals:

Discuss the synergy among nutrition and exercising. Guide readers in putting dietary dreams that complement their fitness objectives, whether or not or not it's miles weight manage, muscle constructing, or preferred health. A nicely-fueled body enables ultimate popular performance.

7. Hydration:

Emphasize the significance of hydration in helping physical hobby. Provide realistic hints for keeping adequate water intake throughout the day and all through exercising sports. Hydration is critical for not unusual fitness and workout common usual overall performance.

eight. Nutrient-Rich Choices:

Encourage a focus on nutrient-dense ingredients that gasoline the body for most reliable everyday performance. Discuss the importance of a properly-balanced weight loss program wealthy in proteins, carbohydrates, fat, vitamins, and minerals. Nutrition performs a vital characteristic in undertaking health dreams.

Prioritizing Recovery:

nine. Sleep and Rest:

Highlight the feature of sleep and rest in the restoration process. Discuss the impact of terrific sleep on time-honored well-being and muscle recovery. Provide techniques for improving sleep hygiene to aid your health adventure.

10. Active Recovery:

Introduce the concept of lively healing. Incorporate light physical sports activities, stretching, or sports activities like yoga on rest days. Emphasize that restoration is an fundamental a part of health development and contributes to ordinary well-being.

Building a Support System:

11. Community Engagement:

Discuss the importance of community engagement, whether or not via network health training, on-line forums, or social media corporations. A supportive network can offer motivation, idea, and a experience of belonging.

12. Accountability Partnerships:

Explore the blessings of duty partnerships. Encourage readers to comprise buddies, own family, or workout buddies to share the adventure, have fun successes, and conquer traumatic conditions collectively.

Reflection and Adaptation:

thirteen. Regular Self-Reflection:

Stress the importance of ordinary self-reflected photo at the health journey. Encourage readers to evaluate progress, have an amazing time achievements, and choose out areas for development. Reflection complements mindfulness and popularity.

14. Adapting Goals:

Discuss the opportunity of adapting health desires based on changing conditions, achievements, or evolving aspirations. Flexibility in goal-setting contributes to sustained motivation and a high-quality thoughts-set.

Designing a sustainable health plan is a pivotal step within the route of prolonged-term success. By balancing sporting activities, prioritizing nutrients, emphasizing recuperation, building a help device, and embracing adaptability, you are developing a framework that is going past exercising—it's far a way of existence. As you embark in this journey, do not forget that each desire contributes for your easy nicely-being.

Here are for your sustained fulfillment and a more healthful, happier you!

Chapter 6: Understanding Functional Fitness

In the Pursuit of Purposeful Movement

1. Definition and Principles of Functional Fitness

Functional fitness embodies a paradigm shift inside the way we technique physical well-being. It's a method rooted within the belief that workout want to now not simplest form our frame but also beautify our capability to move via existence's each day responsibilities effects.

At its essence, beneficial health revolves round actions that mimic real-life activities. It's no longer absolutely about isolated muscle schooling however about integrating various muscle companies to decorate coordination, stability, and common capability. These carrying activities prioritize first-class over quantity, specializing in movement patterns that align with our each day necessities.

The mind of realistic fitness encompasses a mixture of energy, flexibility, stability, and persistence. They are the constructing blocks that red meat up our bodies for the needs of everyday life, nurturing a holistic method to physical properly-being.

2. Explaining the Relevance of Functional Exercises in Daily Life

Consider the smooth act of lifting a grocery bag, playing with children, or maybe sitting down and standing up—

it is in the ones recurring responsibilities in which practical fitness shines. Functional sports activities reflect the ones movements, making prepared our bodies to execute them effectively and without pressure.

Unlike conventional workout routines that isolate muscle tissues or recognition mostly on aesthetics, beneficial sports prioritize movements that translate without delay into our normal sports activities sports. By honing in on those practical movements, we beautify our ability to bend, deliver, push, pull, and twist— moves that outline our each day life.

three. Benefits of Functional Fitness over Traditional Workouts

The superiority of useful health lies not in its complexity however in its practicality. Here's in which it holds a brilliant facet over conventional exercise exercises:

Real-worldwide Application: While traditional exercise exercises frequently purpose specific muscle groups in controlled environments, beneficial fitness thrives on wearing activities that prepare us for actual-international conditions. It's approximately getting organized the frame to function optimally in diverse conditions we stumble upon each day.

Overall Functional Ability: Functional fitness promotes a properly-rounded bodily prowess, now not restricted to muscle duration or energy. It complements mobility, agility, and stability, contributing to a greater resilient frame capable of managing diverse stressful conditions.

Injury Prevention: By strengthening the body as a practical unit, in region of focusing totally on person muscle organizations, beneficial health aids in damage prevention. It addresses weaknesses and imbalances, lowering the hazard of damage subsequently of recurring duties.

Understanding practical health is to consist of a philosophy that extends past the health club. It's approximately nurturing a body able to thriving inside the ebb and go along with the drift of normal life.

In the subsequent chapters, we can delve deeper, exploring checks, foundational sporting activities, and customized sports that encompass the essence of beneficial fitness.

Let's preserve this journey closer to a extra realistic and empowered version humans.

Assessing Your Functional Fitness Level

Mapping Your Path to Functional Proficiency

1. Self-Assessment Tools for Functional Fitness

Before embarking on any health adventure, knowledge in which you stand is crucial. This bankruptcy introduces you to a spectrum of self-evaluation equipment designed to gauge your current diploma of useful health. From clean mobility checks to comparing your power and stability, those device provide a holistic view of your body's useful skills.

These checks are not approximately evaluation but about developing a baseline from which to development. They offer insights into areas that might require interest, guiding you within the route of targeted physical games to decorate your realistic abilities.

2. Understanding Movement Patterns and Identifying Weaknesses

Functional fitness hinges on movement—the ability to perform every day duties with normal overall performance and ease. Understanding your frame's motion patterns is fundamental to unlocking its functionality. By looking the manner you float in the course of regular activities—squatting, bending, lifting—you could pick out any barriers or weaknesses that might beat back your general overall performance.

This financial disaster delves into dissecting movement styles, spotting any asymmetries, imbalances, or hints that would effect your beneficial health. Identifying those weaknesses serves as a compass, guiding you inside the path of wearing events tailor-made to deal with and beautify them.

three. Setting Goals Based on Individual Functional Fitness Needs

With a clear understanding of your cutting-edge purposeful capabilities, it is time to chart a direction in advance. Setting custom designed goals tailored on your specific wishes and aspirations will become the cornerstone of your adventure.

In this segment, we discover the art of purpose putting in the vicinity of practical fitness. Whether it's miles enhancing flexibility, improving middle stability, or building energy for particular activities, those desires function guiding stars, directing your efforts toward tangible and ability results.

By aligning your goals in conjunction with your practical fitness evaluation consequences, you pave the manner for a reason-pushed health routine.

Each reason becomes a stepping stone toward a greater agile, succesful, and practical model of you.

This bankruptcy serves as your compass, guiding you through the initial tiers of your realistic fitness journey. The exams, motion analyses, and goal-putting strategies delivered right here lay the inspiration upon which we're going to bring together as we improvement via the subsequent chapters.

Let's embark in this journey of self-discovery and transformation closer to advanced functional fitness.

Chapter 7: Foundation Exercises for Mobility and Flexibility

Unlocking Fluidity and Range of Motion

1. Warm-up Routines and Dynamic Stretching

The gateway to only mobility and versatility begins offevolved with a properly-designed heat-up habitual. This financial destroy introduces dynamic stretching—an lively shape of stretching that primes the body for motion. Dynamic stretches no longer handiest growth blood go along with the flow and frame temperature but additionally improve joint mobility and muscle elasticity.

Explore a repertoire of dynamic stretches geared toward getting equipped your body for the bodily video games earlier. These movements, performed in motion, serve as a bridge among a sedentary kingdom and an active workout, decreasing the risk of damage and improving regular widespread overall performance.

2. Mobility Exercises for Joints and Muscles

Mobility—the freedom of motion round joints—is a cornerstone of useful health. In this segment, find out a chain of physical sports meticulously curated to enhance joint mobility throughout your frame. These sports goal specific joints and muscle corporations, selling flexibility, balance, and functionality.

From shoulder rotations to hip circles and determination mobility drills, every exercise is designed to beautify the body's natural shape of motion. By incorporating those moves into your routine, you may experience superior flexibility and a extra ease of motion for your each day sports.

3. Flexibility Drills to Improve Range of Motion

Flexibility—the functionality of muscle mass and tendons to prolong—plays a pivotal function in realistic fitness. This segment focuses on flexibility drills geared in the route of enhancing your frame's sort of motion. These drills stretch and prolong muscle groups, considering a broader span of motion with out compromising balance.

Explore quite a few static stretches targeting primary muscle corporations. These stretches, held for period, beneficial aid in lengthening tight muscle groups, growing flexibility, and reducing muscle tension. Embracing the ones drills as a ordinary a part of your habitual fosters superior mobility and flexibility through the years.

This economic catastrophe serves due to the fact the gateway to a greater supple and agile you. By integrating warmth-up sports, dynamic stretching, mobility physical sports activities, and flexibility drills into your regimen, you lay the muse for a frame primed to encompass the stressful conditions and actions of every day life.

Let's embark on this adventure of unlocking your frame's complete capability for fluidity and movement.

Core Strength and Stability

The Foundation of Functional Motion

1. Importance of a Strong Core for Functional Movements

At the coronary coronary coronary heart of each useful motion lies the center—a powerhouse that serves due to the fact the anchor for stability and electricity. This phase illuminates the pivotal role of a robust middle in facilitating ordinary sports activities. Whether it is bending to pick out up groceries, preserving posture in the direction of extended sitting, or undertaking sports activities sports, a sturdy center is essential for executing those actions effectively and minimizing the chance of injury.

Understanding the middle's role as the center of stability and electricity underscores its importance in enhancing normal beneficial fitness. Strengthening the center now not handiest improves physical normal overall performance however additionally contributes to better posture, stability, and spinal fitness.

2. Core-Strengthening Exercises for Stability and Balance

Explore a repertoire of centered carrying sports aimed closer to fortifying your middle muscle organizations. These physical video games embody a spectrum of movements that engage the entire center, which incorporates the abdominals, indirect's, decrease back, and pelvic muscle agencies. From planks and Russian twists to chicken-puppies and leg will increase, every exercise specializes in enhancing stability, stability, and everyday center energy.

This phase offers a entire manual to performing those sports activities with right shape and approach. Mastering the ones moves regularly builds a resilient center, translating into improved stability and stability on your each day sports.

three. Integration of Core Workouts into Daily Routines

Making middle workout workouts a unbroken part of your every day routine is fundamental to reaping their blessings continuously. This phase explores strategies for integrating middle physical games into your regular existence. From incorporating short, centered sports into your morning ordinary to infusing center-strengthening actions into ordinary sports like sitting at a table or watching TV, the ones clean however effective methods make certain that middle strengthening turns into a routine a part of your life-style.

By integrating the ones physical video games into every day existence, you may now not handiest support your middle however furthermore enhance its endurance, contributing to better posture and spinal alignment.

This chapter unveils the significance of a sturdy middle and equips you with the tools to domesticate center power and balance. By embracing center-centered bodily games and seamlessly integrating them into your physical activities, you pave the manner for greater suitable balance, stability, and useful efficiency to your regular movements.

Let's embark on this journey of strengthening the inspiration of your practical fitness via a resilient center.

Functional Strength Training

Empowering Daily Movements with Strength

1. Compound Exercises Targeting Multiple Muscle Groups

Functional energy training revolves spherical compound movements—sporting activities that interact more than one muscle businesses simultaneously. This section unveils the efficacy of compound bodily video games in enhancing everyday power and functionality. Movements like squats, deadlifts, lunges, and push-america of the united states of americaserve as foundational physical activities, mimicking actual-life moves and attractive multiple muscle agencies in a coordinated strive.

By focusing on compound sports activities sports, you no longer amazing optimize your exercise time but also amplify electricity that seamlessly interprets into your normal sports activities.

2. Weight-Bearing Exercises for Functional Strength

Weight-bearing physical video games form the backbone of sensible energy schooling. This phase delves into the importance of the usage of outdoor resistance—whether or no longer via unfastened weights, resistance bands, or body weight—to beautify muscle power and staying strength.

These bodily activities mimic the wishes of every day obligations thru introducing resistance, allowing your muscle mass to comply and develop stronger. By tough your muscle groups in competition to resistance, you foster power that right now contributes for your ability to carry out severa sports activities with out issues.

three. Building Strength for Everyday Activities

The essence of beneficial strength education lies in its realistic application to each day lifestyles. This section specializes in wearing sports specifically designed to decorate power for commonplace every day activities—lifting groceries, sporting youngsters, mountain climbing stairs, or maybe gardening.

Through centered carrying sports tailored to copy those moves, you expand the power essential to navigate the ones sports consequences. By aligning your education with the desires of normal lifestyles, you assemble a body that is not really robust in the fitness center but resilient inside the actual worldwide.

This financial ruin serves as your manual to beneficial energy training—using compound carrying occasions, incorporating weight-bearing wearing events, and fortifying your body for the pains of each day lifestyles. By embracing those sports, you lay the foundation for a more potent, more succesful you.

Let's embark on this journey of cultivating practical power that empowers you to conquer ordinary duties with energy and ease.

Chapter 8: Cardiovascular Endurance for Daily Tasks

Fueling Vitality for Daily Life

1. Cardio Workouts for Enhanced Endurance and Stamina

Cardiovascular health paperwork the cornerstone of practical strength This section illuminates the importance of incorporating aerobic bodily video games to raise your patience and stamina Exercises which includes taking walks, cycling, swimming, and brisk on foot function catalysts in enhancing your cardiovascular health.

These physical games no longer most effective deliver a lift to your coronary coronary heart and lungs however moreover make contributions to superior blood flow into, boosting your potential to hold physical sports at some level in the day.

2. Interval Training and Its Benefits for Daily Life

Explore the transformative power of c language schooling in the realm of practical fitness. This phase sheds slight at the effectiveness of alternating amongst immoderate-intensity bursts and durations of lively recuperation. Interval training not most effective complements cardiovascular patience but moreover mirrors the severa intensity of each day sports.

By simulating the wishes of real-life actions thru durations, you cultivate the capability to address fluctuations in physical attempt, getting ready your frame to conform and carry out optimally all through diverse duties.

3. Incorporating Cardio Exercises into Functional Routines

The essence of purposeful health lies in seamlessly integrating wearing activities into your each day life. This segment makes a speciality of infusing aerobic physical sports into sensible wearing activities. By combining cardiovascular sporting events with movements that mimic every day sports—which includes stair mountaineering, sporting weights, or sporting out agility drills—you create a synergy among cardio health and practical capability.

This integration ensures that your cardiovascular exercising sporting events not handiest beautify staying strength however moreover right now make contributions to your ability to perform everyday responsibilities efficiently.

This chapter serves as a manual to elevating your cardiovascular endurance—a critical element in empowering you to address each day obligations with sustained electricity and resilience. By embracing cardio carrying activities, incorporating interval training, and integrating the ones carrying activities into useful exercises, you pave the manner for higher stamina and strength on your normal existence.

Let's embark in this journey of enhancing your cardiovascular endurance to gasoline your each day pastimes with unwavering power.

Chapter 9: Functional Training for Specific Activities

Empowering Movements for Daily Functionality

1. Tailoring Workouts for Different Daily Tasks (e.G., Lifting, Bending, Carrying)

Functional health is ready making equipped your body for the diverse needs of each day lifestyles. This segment emphasizes the significance of tailoring exercising exercises to align with severa daily obligations. Whether it's far lifting groceries, bending to tie shoelaces, or carrying kids, specific physical video games can replicate and support the muscle mass and movement styles concerned in the ones sports activities.

Explore sports activities that mimic the ones movements, focusing on moves that have interaction the applicable muscle organizations. By tailoring workout physical games to simulate each day obligations, you prepare your body to perform the ones sports activities sports greater correctly and with decreased hazard of strain or harm.

2. Functional Exercises for Common Movements (e.G., Squatting, Pushing, Pulling)

Functional moves are the building blocks of each day sports. This section delves into specific sporting activities that reflect not unusual movements along with squatting, pushing, and pulling. Squats red meat up the lower frame for actions like getting up from a chair, on the same time as pushing and pulling bodily sports decorate better body electricity critical for severa duties.

Discover pretty quite a number sporting sports—body weight, resistance, or beneficial actions—that mimic those moves. These bodily activities goal the muscle corporations and movement styles essential for every day capability, selling power and coordination for the ones vital moves.

three. Injury Prevention via Targeted Functional Training

Functional schooling now not best complements overall performance however moreover plays a essential position in damage prevention. This segment specializes in targeted functional training to lessen the risk of accidents for the duration of every day activities. By strengthening muscular tissues and enhancing mobility in precise areas prone to harm, you create a protective protect in opposition to ability damage.

By emphasizing proper form, muscle balance, and joint balance in practical sports activities, you mitigate the hazard of lines and accidents all through everyday duties. Incorporating those sports into your regular promotes longevity and sustained functionality.

This bankruptcy serves as your guide to tailoring sports activities, gaining knowledge of common moves, and preventing injuries through targeted functional education. By getting prepared your body for the unique wishes of each day lifestyles, you cultivate resilience, power, and damage resistance.

Let's embark on this adventure of empowering your frame to excel inside the day by day sports that outline your lifestyles.

Integrating Functional Fitness into Daily Routine

Crafting a Lifestyle of Functional Vitality

1. Creating a Personalized Functional Fitness Plan

Your adventure inside the path of useful health starts offevolved with a customised plan tailored on your desires and aspirations. This phase courses you through the technique of crafting a useful health plan. Assess your desires, keep in thoughts your contemporary-day health diploma, and choose out sports that align together collectively along with your manner of existence and alternatives.

By outlining a plan that consists of sports activities focused on mobility, energy, staying strength, and versatility, you lay the basis for an entire and doable ordinary.

2. Tips for Staying Motivated and Consistent

Consistency is fundamental in any fitness enterprise. This phase gives insights and techniques to live inspired and devoted for your beneficial fitness adventure. Explore techniques inclusive of setting realistic goals, monitoring development, finding a workout buddy, or incorporating rewards to keep your motivation levels excessive.

Additionally, find out the strength of variety to your workouts. Incorporating unique sporting occasions, attempting new sports activities sports, or editing your ordinary periodically can maintain your wearing activities fresh and attractive.

three. Adapting Exercises to Fit Busy Lifestyles

This segment explores practical hints and strategies for adapting physical games to in shape busy schedules. Whether it's miles breaking bodily games into shorter, greater conceivable sessions or incorporating sensible sporting sports into ordinary obligations, find out strategies to seamlessly integrate health into your each day lifestyles.

By exploring time-saving strategies, prioritizing exercise workouts, and making fitness an crucial a part of your recurring, you make sure that beneficial health becomes a sustainable way of existence desire.

This bankruptcy serves as your guide to seamlessly integrating sensible health into your every day ordinary. By developing a custom designed plan, staying influenced and ordinary, and adapting wearing sports activities to fit your busy manner of life, you pave the way for a way of existence brimming with power and capability.

Let's embark in this adventure of embedding useful fitness into the fabric of your each day lifestyles.

Nutrition and Recovery for Functional Fitness

Nourishment and Rejuvenation for Optimal Performance

1. Importance of Proper Nutrition for Functional Fitness

Nutrition office work the inspiration upon which beneficial fitness flourishes. This phase emphasizes the crucial position of proper vitamins in assisting your realistic fitness goals. A well-balanced healthy eating plan wealthy in vitamins fuels your sports activities, aids in muscle healing, and sustains your body's energy levels.

Explore the significance of macronutrients (proteins, carbohydrates, and fats) and micronutrients (nutrients and minerals) in assisting your body's sensible demands. Understanding how meals serves as gas for your workout routines and aids in muscle restore and increase is pivotal in optimizing your health journey.

2. Post-Workout Recovery Strategies

Recovery is as critical due to the fact the workout itself in a purposeful health regimen. This segment delves into effective post-exercising recovery strategies aimed towards optimizing your body's recuperative strategies. Explore techniques which includes proper hydration, adequate sleep, foam rolling, and stretching to lessen muscle pain and decorate recovery.

Understanding the significance of healing lets in your frame to adapt to the stresses of workout, selling muscle repair and boom, and ensuring sustained basic overall performance.

3. Balancing Diet to Support Functional Fitness Goals

Tailoring your weight loss plan to align together in conjunction with your functional fitness dreams is paramount. This segment navigates the intricacies of balancing your healthy dietweight-reduction plan to assist your specific fitness goals. Whether it's preserving a caloric stability, timing your food spherical physical games, or emphasizing nutrient-dense components, discover dietary strategies that supplement your beneficial health goals.

By optimizing your weight loss plan to fuel your workout exercises, resource in restoration, and assist muscle growth and restore, you beautify the effectiveness of your practical fitness recurring.

This financial disaster serves as your guide to leveraging vitamins and healing strategies to extend the benefits of beneficial fitness. By embracing right nutrition, implementing effective put up-exercise recovery strategies, and balancing your weight loss plan to assist your health goals, you lay the basis for a nourished and rejuvenated frame geared for max useful ordinary common overall performance.

Let's embark in this adventure of nourishing and revitalizing your body for top beneficial fitness.

Beyond the Book: Long-Term Functional Fitness

Embracing a Lifestyle of Lasting Vitality

1. Sustaining Progress and Continual Improvement

The adventure of practical health extends some distance beyond the pages of this ebook. Sustaining improvement calls for a willpower to persistent development. This section explores strategies for preserving and advancing your useful health tiers. Set new desires, diversify your sports activities, and continuously mission your body to evolve and grow.

By embracing the mind-set of non-stop improvement, you make certain that realistic fitness remains an evolving adventure, now not a holiday spot reached.

2. Seeking Professional Guidance and Community Support

Navigating the complexities of health regularly advantages from professional steerage and network aid. This section highlights the significance of looking for assist from health professionals, running shoes, or coaches who concentrate on beneficial fitness. Their facts can provide personalized steerage, deal with particular issues, and splendid-music your wearing activities for maximum beneficial consequences.

Furthermore, locating a network or aid community of individuals pursuing comparable health dreams can offer encouragement, obligation, and shared reviews. Engaging with like-minded human beings fosters motivation and crew spirit in your health adventure.

3. Embracing Functional Fitness as a Lifestyle Choice

Functional health transcends an insignificant exercising recurring; it embodies a holistic way of lifestyles preference. This phase emphasizes the mixing of practical fitness into your each day lifestyles beyond scheduled exercising exercises. Whether it is adopting energetic pastimes, choosing motion-wealthy sports, or retaining mindfulness approximately movement patterns, realistic fitness becomes an intrinsic part of how you stay and drift.

By embracing practical health as a way of lifestyles desire, you no longer most effective maintain your physical earnings however also enhance your standard nicely-being, improving your pleasant of lifestyles.

This financial disaster serves as a manual to embracing the extended-term components of useful fitness—a self-control to continual improvement, searching out expert steering and community assist, and integrating functional health as a way of life preference. By adopting those standards, you pave the manner for sustained energy and capability throughout your life.

www.ingramcontent.com/pod-product-compliance
Lightning Source LLC
Chambersburg PA
CBHW051726020426
42333CB00014B/1174